Combat Nutrition

Military-inspired Fitness and Recovery Foods

Table of Contents

Chapter 1. Introduction

Welcome to an invigorating journey through the battle-hardened world of Combat Nutrition: Military-inspired Fitness and Recovery Foods! This Special Report not only dives deep into the hearty grub and energy-packed elixirs that fuel our brave troops, but it also examines the science behind these nutritional strategies. These soldier-tested, expert-approved dietary plans are not just for the battlefield but also for your everyday life. They have the power to boost your fitness regime, enhance recovery, and turn you into a wellness warrior! So get ready to embark on this thrilling quest –absorb the wisdom, implement the tactics, and conquer your fitness goals. Can anyone resist the call to be as fit, mentally tough and resilient as our military heroes? Buy this Special Report and start your transformation today!

Chapter 2. An Overview of Combat Nutrition

Before diving into the deeper aspects of combat nutrition, it's essential to understand the overarching principles. The diets of military personnel, especially those who serve during duty overseas or in special operations, are intended to meet high energy demands and promote optimal performance while considering factors like portability, shelf-life, and taste.

At its core, combat nutrition revolves around three main components—macronutrients, micronutrients, and hydration. Each component plays a pivotal role in ensuring soldiers are at their physical and mental peak, ready to tackle any challenges on the battlefield.

2.1. Macronutrients

Macronutrients include proteins, carbohydrates, and fats. All these are key to sustaining energy, building and repairing muscle tissue, and supporting healthy cognitive function.

1. *Protein:* Serving both as a fuel source and a building block to repair and grow tissues, protein is the centerpiece of combat nutrition. Soldiers typically need to consume more protein than civilians do because of the intense muscular stress they undergo. In addition to meats, protein can be found in eggs, nuts, seeds, and legumes.

2. *Carbohydrates:* Carbohydrates are the body's primary energy source. Complex carbs, like those found in whole grains, vegetables, and legumes, are preferred over simple carbs due to their sustained energy release pattern. Pre-packaged meals for soldiers, known as Meals, Ready-to-Eat (MRE), often comprise of a

high percentage of carbohydrates due to their energy-rich nature.

3. *Fats:* Fats are a dense energy source, providing more than twice the energy per gram than proteins or carbs. Fats are also essential for absorbing micronutrients and maintaining core body temperature. Healthy fats include polyunsaturated fats like omega-3, which aids brain function and reduces inflammation, found in sources like fish, nuts, and seeds.

2.2. Micronutrients

While they're required in smaller amounts, micronutrients—vitamins and minerals—are critical for a multitude of bodily functions, including bolstering the immune system, enhancing wound healing ability, and protecting against oxidative damage. Each MRE is designed to provide a soldier with one-third of his or her required daily intake of essential vitamins and minerals.

1. *Vitamins:* Particularly, B vitamins help the body to metabolize food for energy, while Vitamin C and E are powerful antioxidants. On the other hand, vitamin D, obtainable through sun exposure, plays a vital role in maintaining bone health.

2. *Minerals:* Essential minerals include iron for transporting oxygen in blood, calcium for bone health and nerve function, zinc for wound healing, and magnesium for protein synthesis.

2.3. Hydration

Hydration is the final pillar of combat nutrition. Whether on a desert patrol or performing a high-altitude jump, servicemen and women must stay adequately hydrated to maintain overall health and performance. Dehydration can lead to fatigue, dizziness, and decreased cognitive performance, all of which are detrimental in a combat environment.

Gone are the days where water was the only hydration option. Modern military forces around the world use rehydration solutions containing electrolytes and carbohydrates to improve fluid absorption and preserve energy levels. Electrolytes—like sodium, potassium, and chloride—maintain fluid balance in the body and are essential for muscle and nerve function.

2.4. Combat Rations: The Backbone of Soldier Nutrition

Combat rations, colloquially known as rat packs, are the primary way soldiers receive their food in the field. They often come in lightweight, compact, all-in-one meal packs, and are constructed to withstand adverse conditions and have extended shelf lives.

An MRE, for instance, typically comprises an energy-dense main meal, a snack, some form of drink mix or electrolyte powder, and a dessert. The contents are designed to be eaten on the go or prepared with minimal equipment in a variety of environments, all while providing a balanced nutrition profile for a soldier.

The evolution of combat rations has seen the incorporation of more varied dietary needs, improved taste profiles, and addition of functional items like caffeinated gum for temporary alertness or tubes of peanut butter for a quick energy boost.

2.5. Tailoring Nutrition to the Mission

The specific nutritional requirement of military personnel can vary significantly depending on their role, gender, age, the environmental conditions they're operating in, and the physical demands of their mission. Therefore, nutrition in the military is a dynamic regime that requires careful consideration and timely adjustments.

A physically demanding role might necessitate a higher intake of protein and carbohydrates to support muscle recovery and maintain energy levels. Likewise, operating in a colder climate might call for an increased caloric intake to compensate for the additional energy expended in preserving body heat.

2.6. Nutrition for Productivity and Mental Vigour

The field of combat nutrition extends beyond physical performance—it's also deeply intertwined with cognitive performance. Maintaining focus, decision-making ability, memory, and response time under extreme stress involves consuming adequate amounts of specific nutrients like carbohydrates, omega-3 fats, and certain vitamins and minerals.

Moreover, nutrition plays a vital role in managing the psychological stresses of military life. Dietary strategies can help regulate mood and sleep, key variables in maintaining mental health and resilience.

Indeed, the science of combat nutrition has evolved into much more than just "eating enough to stay alive." It's a sophisticated, meticulously crafted science that empowers our troops to operate at the zenith of their potential—physically and mentally. Above all, it's about fueling the soldier's body and soul under some of the most challenging, harrowing circumstances imaginable. Armed with knowledge on the principles of combat nutrition, you're now ready to delve deeper into this fascinating field.

Chapter 3. The Science behind Military-Grade Fitness

Understanding the rigorous physical demands of military personnel helps us decode the role of nutrition in keeping them fit, focused, and ready for the call of duty. These men and women are often subjected to strenuous exercise, extreme weather, inadequate sleep, psychological stress, and lack of healthy food and water, all of which put extreme demands on their health. The science of military-grade fitness nutrition hinges on key principles that address these unique challenges, promoting endurance, strength, recovery, and mental tenacity.

3.1. Basics of Combat Nutrition

At the heart of combat nutrition is the understanding of biochemical reactions in the body. Carbohydrates, proteins, and fats—the three primary macronutrients—are vital for optimum physical and mental performance. Carbohydrates are the body's primary energy source, while proteins support muscle repair and growth. Fats, although demonized, also play a key role, providing concentrated energy and facilitating vitamin absorption and hormonal regulation.

3.2. Impact of Exercise on the Body

Physical activity fuels the demand for nutrients. As exercise increases in intensity, the need for carbohydrates escalates due to the body's usage of glycogen, a stored form of glucose. Therefore, soldiers are instructed to consume carb-rich meals before engaging in strenuous activities to maintain energy levels. Similarly, high-protein foods post-exercise aid in muscle recovery and rebuilding.

3.3. The Importance of Hydration

Maintaining hydration is essential in military nutrition. The body's fluid balance is critical for regulating body temperature, ensuring muscle function, and facilitating nutrient transport. Dehydration poses a serious health risk that can impair physical performance and cognitive function. Thus, drinking water and replenishing electrolytes is emphasized during and after workouts.

3.4. Caloric Deficit: A Common Challenge

Military personnel often face caloric deficits due to increased physical activity and limited meal times. It's crucial to address this, as prolonged inadequate energy intake can lead to fat loss, muscle wasting, and decreased physical performance. Soldiers are encouraged to carry energy-dense, nutrient-rich snacks to help overcome this deficit.

3.5. Harnessing the Power of Micronutrients

Though macronutrients form the base of combat nutrition, micronutrients play equally valuable roles. Vitamins and minerals aid in energy production, oxygen transport, bone formation, and immune defense. Supplementing these can bridge dietary gaps and ensure optimal nutrient intake.

3.6. Importance of Meal Timing

Eating at the right time—and resting—can amplify performance and recovery. Pre-exercise meals rich in carbs and protein can provide energy. Replenishing nutrients after training aids in repairing tissues and refilling glycogen stores. Adequate rest is equally crucial, as it allows the body to recover, adapt and build strength for future tasks.

3.7. Mental Resilience and Nutrition

Combat readiness isn't just about the body—it involves mental resilience too. Omega-3 fatty acids, found in fatty fish and chia seeds, support brain function and mental well-being. Nutrients like B-vitamins, iron, iodine, and zinc also contribute to cognitive health, improving attention, memory, and decision-making abilities.

3.8. Tailored Nutrition Plans

"The one-size-fits-all" approach doesn't work with military nutrition. Individually tailored plans, considering factors like age, gender, health status, and activity levels, are essential for maximal fitness and recovery. Each soldier's nutritional needs and challenges are unique and should be adjusted accordingly.

3.9. Keeping Pace with Technological Advances

As technology evolves, so does the science of military nutrition. Innovative solutions like portable nutrient-dense meals, advanced hydration strategies, and precision nutrition, unveiled through wearable tech and genetic profiling, are transforming the battlefield, enabling soldiers to stay physically and mentally sharp.

Adopting these combat nutrition strategies isn't just for military personnel. They're valuable for anyone looking to improve physical performance, speed up recovery, and promote overall health. By understanding and integrating these principles, you're charting a powerful blueprint for fitness success, one that keeps you resilient in the face of challenges—just like a soldier on the battlefield.

Chapter 4. Fueling the Forces: Diet Strategy and its Evolution

Despite often being overlooked, the role of nutrition in military operations dates back to the earliest recorded battles in history. Understanding the evolution of dietary strategies in the military provides insight into today's nutritional requirements for our troops and, in turn, can potentially contribute to enhancing fitness regimes and recovery capabilities for civilians as well.

4.1. The Ancient and Medieval Age: Early Approaches to Combat Nutrition

In the classical ages, armies mainly subsisted on staple foods. For Roman legions, for example, the diet was predominantly grain-based. The daily ration was about two pounds of grain, either in the form of bread or porridge. In contrast, the Greeks were known to consume a concoction of vinegar and water called "posca" that aided hydration. Soldiers also ate meat, olive oil, and wine to provide a wider range of nutrients.

Medieval armies had a typical diet that included bread, dried fruits, some sort of protein in the form of preserved meats or cheese, and beer or wine. Knights and higher-ranking officials had better access to fresh food and meat. Nutrition, while fundamental, was often secondary to logistical challenges; the primary concern was getting adequate food supplies to the soldiers.

4.2. The Discovery of Vitamins and the Start of Modern Combat Nutrition

The 18th and 19th centuries marked significant turning points in combat nutrition. For one, the discovery of vitamins began to underscore the importance of a balanced diet. The problem of scurvy among sailors was solved with the introduction of lime juice, rich in Vitamin C. This marked one of the first application of nutritional science in the military.

In the American Civil War, soldiers generally ate hardtack, a type of dense biscuit, along with salt pork and coffee. While the diet was hearty, it lacked vital nutrients. As a result of these nutrition shortfalls, many soldiers fell ill due to malnutrition rather than their wounds.

4.3. Military Nutrition in the World Wars

During World War I and II, there was an even greater understanding of the role of nutrition in maintaining soldier health and enhancing performance. Governments began to invest more in research to perfect the diets of the soldiers.

In World War I, soldiers received canned meat (known as bully beef), hardtack biscuits, and tea with sugar. There were also fruits and jam to add a bit of variety. During World War II, the US introduced the K-ration, a daily food ration initially intended for paratroopers consisting of a mix of balanced foods. The evolution of the canned food technologies during the WWI also improved the quality, safety and longevity of foods in war times.

4.4. Today's Combat Nutrition: A Catered Approach

Modern combat nutrition has come a long way. The US Military, for example, has a range of meals ready to eat (MREs) designed specifically with the nutrient requirements of combat troops in mind. These meals contain a balance of carbohydrates, protein, fat, as well as key vitamins and minerals. Furthermore, there is a greater emphasis on hydration, with energy drinks being an essential part of a soldier's kit.

Nutritionists are now part of a soldier's training staff, providing personalized advice to optimize performance. There's also a focus on nutritional supplementation, including vitamins, protein bars, and recovery shakes, to meet the rigorous physical demands placed on modern soldiers.

4.5. How This Applies To Your Everyday Life

The military's evolution of combat nutrition offers valuable lessons for individuals pursuing their own fitness goals. The balance of macronutrients (carbohydrates, protein, fat) and the increased focus on hydration display an effective strategy for energy and recovery.

While average civilians may not experience the same harsh environments or demanding physical exertion as those in military training, adopting a military-inspired approach to nutrition can help attain optimal performance and improved recovery time.

By focusing on a balanced diet that meets your personal macro and micronutrient requirements, staying sufficiently hydrated, and potentially augmenting your diet with appropriate supplements, you can revise your diet strategy to mimic the effectiveness of our modern forces.

The comprehension of combat nutrition's evolution enables us to better conceptualize the importance of appropriately fueling our bodies according to our individual activities and goals. With lessons taken from battlefield to boardroom, the potential to elevate your performance and recovery is within reach.

Chapter 5. Power Foods: Energy Optimization for Peak Performance

Keeping a sharp mind and a robust body is non-negotiable for soldiers. Meeting this requirement is a challenge in itself, but when you add the elements of extreme environments and brutal workouts to the mix, the difficulty level soars high. The secret to this herculean task of maintaining peak physical prowess could be hidden in plain sight, on our plates – the power foods.

Empowering our military heroes and now, warranting your attention as well, these power foods are not just your average meals. These are energy-optimized, performance-enhancing dietary champions that boost strength, endurance, and speed up recovery.

5.1. The Science Behind Fuel

Before you embark on this nutritional journey, it's crucial to understand what 'fuel' means for your body. Energy-yielding nutrients—carbohydrates, fats, and proteins—are the stars of this show. They each play a role yet have diverging paths to contribute energy.

Carbohydrates, available as sugars, starches, and fibers, are your body's primary energy source. They assist in fueling your brain and muscles during physical activity.

Proteins, made up of amino acids, are vital for repairing and building tissue, producing enzymes and hormones, and aiding in immune function.

Fats, often demonized, are actually critical for various bodily functions like vitamin and mineral absorption, and providing concentrated energy.

5.2. Carbohydrates: The First Line of Defense

Food	Carbohydrates (per 100g)	Calories
Oatmeal	66g	389
Brown Rice	77g	370
Sweet Potatoes	20g	86
Quinoa	64g	368

These complex carbohydrates provide a slow, steady release of energy making them an ideal choice for sustained intensity activities that our military heroes regularly undertake.

Taken before a workout, they prevent muscle glycogen depletion, allowing you to work out longer. Post-workout, they replenish glycogen stores and restore energy levels.

5.3. Powering Through with Protein

Food	Protein (per 100g)	Calories
Chicken Breast	31g	165
Tuna	26g	132
Greek Yogurt	10g	59
Almonds	21g	579

Protein is crucial for muscle repair and growth, and it also plays a vital role in promoting satiety and fat loss. Consuming adequate protein ensures that the body maintains lean muscle and assists with recovery post-exercise.

5.4. The Prominence of Fats

Food	Fats (per 100g)	Calories
Avocado	15g	160
Almonds	50g	579
Salmon	13g	206
Olive Oil	100g	884

Fats, particularly unsaturated fats, are essential for hormone production, brain health, and providing energy, particularly for low-intensity, long-duration activities.

5.5. The Magic of Micronutrients

Besides macronutrients, maintaining peak performance requires a plethora of vitamins and minerals essential for various body functions, from energy production to immune health.

Food	Key Micronutrients	Spinach
Iron, Vitamins A, C and K	Bell Peppers	Vitamin C
Whole Eggs	Vitamin B12, Selenium	Bananas

Remember, it's about combining these power foods to create fuel-intense meals that work best for you. Smart nutrition is about setting the stage for sustained energy delivery, keeping muscles in prime working condition, and ensuring optimal recovery after intense training. Stick to these principles, and like our military heroes, you too will conquer whatever physical challenges life throws at you.

Chapter 6. Lessons from the Battlefield: Recovery Foods and Techniques

The invaluable lessons garnered from battlefield canteens provide a unique window into robust dietary strategies that are pivotal in the recovery process. These practical insights derived from combat zones can be harnessed to accelerate recovery and catapult your fitness levels to new heights.

6.1. Feeding the Frontline: The Integral Role of Nutrition in Recovery

In a high-stress environment like the battlefield, ensuring optimal nutrition is crucial. Provisions for troops are carefully selected to provide the best balance of nutrients — a mix that complements the challenging physical activities and aids rapid recovery and healing. Incorporating these strategies into your everyday dietary regime can jump-start your post-exercise recovery and help your body bounce back faster after strenuous workouts.

Diet is the first line of defense when it comes to recovery. Beyond mending the body, the right kind of fuel positively affects your mood, stamina, and resilience, key aspects that often need to be replenished after intense activity. A strategic blend of proteins, carbohydrates, and fats forms the bedrock of this health-boosting military-inspired nutritional plan.

6.2. Protein: The Building Blocks of Recovery

Protein needs little introduction as a major player in recovery. The amino acids that constitute protein are the foundation blocks for repairing and building new muscle tissues. Moreover, these nutrients kick-start the healing process by reducing the concentration of the stress hormone, cortisol, in our system.

Protein recommendations for soldiers typically exceed the average daily requirements due to their demanding physical exertions. This principle is commonplace in the athletic world, too — it's advisable to consume approximately 1.2-2 grams of protein per kilogram of body weight daily, depending on the intensity and frequency of workouts. Incorporating enough protein in your diet not only expedites the recovery process but also helps maintain muscle mass and strength.

Chicken, turkey, beans, legumes, and eggs are excellent protein sources you could integrate into your diet for recovery. Vegan or vegetarian? No problem! Quinoa, tofu, lentils, and tempeh are just as great. However, it's crucial to split protein intake throughout the day rather than pile it all onto one meal. This optimizes the absorption of these essential nutrients by your body.

6.3. Carbohydrates: The Energy Restorers

The next key component in a military-inspired recovery diet is carbohydrates. Contrary to popular diet fads, carbohydrates are not the enemy; instead, they're an ally in recovery. Carbs replenish the glycogen stores in your muscles, depleted during strenuous workouts, and provide the energy required for muscle repair.

Think of carbohydrates intake like a petrol tank: it needs to be refilled after prolonged use. This is why soldiers' meals are typically high in carbohydrates — they're designed to provide sufficient fuel to keep the body going. The choice of carbohydrates matters, too. Focus on complex carbs like oats, brown rice, whole wheat bread, and starchy vegetables. These sources provide a steady stream of energy rather than sudden spikes, ensuring sustained recovery.

6.4. Fats: The Unsung Heroes

In the military dietary playbook, fats also play a crucial part. As energy-dense nutrients, they're essential in refueling the body. They aid in the absorption of fat-soluble vitamins, contribute to hormone production, and serve as a long-term energy reserve. Fats are particularly instrumental in tackling exhaustive missions that last several days, where energy expenditure significantly exceeds intake.

When integrating fats into your recovery diet, opt for sources of unsaturated fats like avocados, salmon, nuts, and seeds. These foods promote heart health, control blood sugar levels, and reduce inflammation — a common aftermath of tough workouts.

6.5. Hydration: Unleashing the Power of Water

Hydration is another pivotal piece of the nutrition puzzle, often overlooked in standard recovery plans. In high-intensity exercises or combat situations, the body can lose significant amounts of water through sweat. This leads to dehydration, which compromises your body's ability to regulate temperature, maintain blood volume, and facilitate recovery.

Water is not just essential for hydration but also for energy production, nutrient transportation, and flushing toxins out of the body. Even a 2% drop in hydration can have detrimental effects on physical performance, cognitive abilities, and mood. To keep your body operating optimally, aim to drink at least 8-10 glasses of water a day, and more if your workouts are intense or you spend much time outdoors.

6.6. Micronutrients: The Invisible Strength-Boosters

While our focus often remains on macros, we cannot overlook the importance of micronutrients in post-workout recovery. Zinc, Iron, Vitamins A, C, and E, and B-Vitamins play a critical role in energy production, red blood cell creation, immune function, and muscle repair.

Fruits and vegetables, dairy, legumes, nuts, seeds, and lean meats are stocked with these micronutrients. Integrating these into your diet can notably enhance your body's recovery and readiness for future activity.

6.7. Conclusion: Tailoring Battle-tested Strategies to Personal Needs

While adopting these military-inspired techniques, remember that recovery isn't a one-size-fits-all process. There's immense value in customizing these strategies based on your unique needs, fitness goals, lifestyle, and personal tastes. Nutrition, after all, should be a marriage of health and pleasure.

Fuel your body like a soldier, respect its need for recovery, and watch as it rewards you with enhanced performance, resilience, and overall wellness. Embrace this nutritional quest unflinchingly, just as the brave troops do on the battlefield, and charge forth to conquer your fitness aspirations!

Chapter 7. Unveiling the Military Nutrition Pyramid

An excellent approach to understanding the components of military nutrition is to visualize it as a pyramid. The Military Nutrition Pyramid demonstrates that not all foods are created equal and directs individuals on how to use these variations to power their optimum performance.

7.1. The Base - Macros: Protons, Carbohydrates, Fats

The foundation of the Military Nutrition Pyramid is comprised of the macronutrients: Proteins, Carbohydrates, and Fats. These Macronutrients form the base as they provide the body with the energy it needs to perform at peak levels.

Most meals should primarily consist of carbohydrates - between 45% to 65% of total caloric intake. Proteins, on the other hand, should constitute 10% to 35%, while fats should make up 20% to 35%.

Carbohydrates are the body's primary energy source as they are easily converted into glucose, which fuels the muscles and brain. Protein is valuable for repairing and rebuilding body tissues, especially after strenuous activities. Fats are vital for hormonal production, insulation, and offering a backup energy source when carbohydrate stores are depleted. Remember, it's important to focus on healthy sources like complex carbohydrates, lean proteins, and unsaturated fats for your macronutrients.

7.2. The Second Tier - Micronutrients: Vitamins and Minerals

The second tier of the pyramid focuses on micronutrients: essential vitamins and minerals. While micro in nature, these nutrients play macro roles in the body's overall performance and recovery. They are required in smaller quantities but are crucial for energy production, bone health, immunity, and repair.

Include a variety of fruits, vegetables, lean meats, dairy, and whole grains in your diet to ensure you're obtaining an array of micronutrients. Some key vitamins and minerals include calcium for strong bones, iron for oxygen transport, and vitamins A, C, and E for robust immunity.

7.3. The Third Tier - Hydration: Water and Electrolytes

Just above micronutrients is hydration, specifically water and electrolytes. Staying adequately hydrated is fundamental to performance as even slight dehydration can impair physical and cognitive functions. For military personnel undergoing intense physical activity and operating in environments where the temperature may fluctuate drastically, hydration cannot be understated.

Water helps in temperature regulation, waste removal, and nutrient transport. Meanwhile, electrolytes (like sodium and potassium) help maintain fluid balance and healthy muscle contractions. Around 3.7 liters of fluids for men and 2.7 liters for women daily is generally recommended. However, these amounts should be increased with exercise and warmer weather.

7.4. The Fourth Tier - Pre-and-Post-Exercise Nutrition

Pre-and-post-exercise nutrition is something special to those doing high-intensity activities like the military. This tier equips individuals with the necessary fuel before an intense workout and supplies needed nutrients for recovery post-workout.

About 1-4 hours before an intense activity, consume a combination of easily digestible carbohydrates and protein, for example, a banana with low-fat Greek yogurt. This provides fuel and helps preserve muscle mass. Within 30 minutes to 2 hours post-workout, refuel with a similar combination to restore glycogen stores and assist in muscle recovery.

7.5. The Apex - Supplements

The apex of the Military Nutrition Pyramid represents supplements - these can fill the nutrient gaps and boost particular areas like muscle recovery or energy production. Although, it's crucial to recognize that supplements should never replace a balanced diet. They are additions, not substitutes.

Common supplements include multivitamins, fish oil for omega-3 fatty acids, branched-chain amino acids (BCAAs) for muscle recovery, and caffeine for enhanced alertness and performance. Remember, always consult with a healthcare provider before adding a new supplement to your regimen.

7.6. Anchoring all Tiers - Consistency

Blanketing all levels of the pyramid is consistency. Consistent good habits become lifestyle, and this is what makes the Military Nutrition Pyramid sustainable. Stick to your dietary plan, stay hydrated, and ensure you're meeting your nutritional needs daily.

In conclusion, the Military Nutrition Pyramid is not just a diet plan, but a comprehensive lifestyle approach. It encourages balanced macro and micronutrient intake, emphasizes hydration, provides guidance for pre-and-post-exercise nutrition, and considers the strategic use of supplements, all under the umbrella of consistency. By incorporating these principles, you can elevate your regimen, enhancing performance, and gaining the resilience of a wellness warrior.

Chapter 8. Real-Life Success Stories: Tales from the Trenches

For as long as remembered, military personnel have been held as epitomes of grit, resilience, and endurance. Understandably, their triumphs are not just about their training and fitness, but also about their nutritional strategies. This curated selection of real-life success stories will not only inspire you, but also provide you with practical insights into incorporating military-style nutrition and fitness into your lifestyle.

8.1. The Long-distance Marine: Sgt. Jake Robinson

Jake Robinson, a marine sergeant, is a testament to the limitless potential of military-grade endurance. For Robinson, running a marathon wasn't a big deal, and neither was a 50 mile ultra-marathon. His real test was the formidable Western States 100-mile endurance run, known as one of the toughest foot races in the world.

Robinson's secret wasn't just his training regime, but also his replenishment strategy. He consumed a steady stream of balanced, complex carbohydrates — oatmeal, sweet potatoes, and wholegrain pastas — at every meal. Before each long run, he would have a hearty serving of slow-release carbs to maintain energy levels. Supplementing this, he ingested military-grade protein shakes immediately after every training session to kickstart his recovery process.

8.2. From the Air Force to CrossFit Competitor: Lt. Olivia Banner

Next on our list is Lt. Olivia Banner, an incredibly fit member of the Air Force who later became a CrossFit competitor. Banner's nutritional strategy differed considerably from Robinson's. She tailored her diet to her rigorous CrossFit routine, which required quick bursts of energy.

Banner incorporated more high-quality fats into her diet, such as avocados, oily fish, and nuts. They not only provided her with immediate and sustained energy but also aided her repair and recovery process. She also implemented an intermittent fasting strategy that aligned well with her military discipline. This provided her body with a regular reset, helping her to stay lean and perform optimally.

8.3. The Infantryman's Recovery: Pvt. Harrison Reed

Private Harrison Reed, an infantryman who suffered a serious injury during training, faced a long and arduous recovery process. For Reed, nutrition became a cornerstone during his rehabilitation journey.

Reed was given a high-protein diet, brimming with lean meats, dairy, legumes, and protein supplements. The purpose was to equip his body with the building blocks needed to repair damaged tissues and muscles. Simultaneously, his diet was fortified with certain micronutrients, like Vitamin C, to facilitate connective tissue repair and Vitamin D to enhance bone strength.

8.4. The Commando's Mental Tonic: Cpt. Ethan James

Lastly, let's look at Captain Ethan James, an elite commando known for his mental stamina. Part of the secret behind James' unflappable mental fortitude was his diet. He adhered strictly to a diet rich in Omega-3 fatty acids from fatty fish, nuts, and seeds and choline from eggs and lean meats. These nutrients, studied for their brain health benefits, improved his mental acuity.

Each of these individuals showcase how key principles of military nutrition translate to various realms of fitness and recovery. Their stories reveal that anyone can experience the benefits of this combat-ready diet, whether they're looking to run longer, perform better in high-intensity workouts, recover from injury, or sharpen their mental edge. Quintessentially, the power of military-backed nutrition can help you attain a fighting-fit life, regardless of the trenches you need to traverse.

Chapter 9. Bridging the Gap: From Soldiers to Civilians

Understanding the difference in nutritional requirements between soldiers and civilians is crucial. This gap is more extensive than you might think, given the significant differences between the physical and mental demands placed on military personnel compared to the average person. In this chapter, we will explore the essential aspects of combat nutrition, and how civilians can adapt these to their everyday lives to enhance health, fitness, and resilience.

9.1. Soldier vs. Civilian: The Primary Differences

Soldiers operate in harsh environments, carrying heavy loads over long distances, under the constant threat of combat. Their bodies are thus subjected to immense physical and mental stress, necessitating a different level of nutrition. Unlike the average civilian who mostly engages in moderate daily activities, soldiers need energy-rich foods that can quickly replenish depleted energy reserves. This means high-protein, high-carb, and high-fat meals are essential, alongside vitamins, minerals, and antioxidants to ward off disease and injury.

Although the majority of civilians do not endure such extreme conditions, certain elements of the military diet can enhance civilians' vitality, fitness, and overall well-being. Additionally, those involved in high-intensity fitness programs can similarly benefit from such a nutrient-dense, high-calorie diet to fuel their workouts.

Chapter 10. Nutrition Strategies for Civilians

10.1. Adapting Combat Nutrition Strategies

First and foremost, the diet should be adapted to individual needs depending on the level of physical activity, age, sex and health condition. However, among the strategies that civilians could adopt from military nutrition are: ingesting protein-packed meals to fuel muscle growth and recovery, consuming complex carbs for sustained energy, and eating healthy fats to support overall health, mood, and brain function.

Adjusting portion sizes is also essential. As civilians typically require fewer calories than soldiers, portion control is vital to prevent over-consumption and weight gain.

10.2. Hydration as a Key Element

Water is the underappreciated hero in nutrition. It lubricates joints, aids digestion, works to regulate body temperature, and helps transport nutrients to various parts of the body. It's no surprise, then, that staying hydrated is a top priority for soldiers.

For civilians, adequate water consumption is also essential. The general recommendation is eight 8-ounce glasses per day, although this can vary. Those involved in intense physical activities may need more, similar to soldiers in active duty.

10.3. Supplements for Enhanced Performance

Supplement usage is common among soldiers to boost performance, recovery, and overall health. Civilians, particularly those involved in strenuous fitness regimens, can adopt this practice, albeit carefully. Nutritional supplementation should only accompany a balanced diet, not replace it.

10.4. Meal Timing and Frequency

In the military world, the saying "eat when you can" is often heard due to the unpredictable nature of field operations. Soldiers are taught to make use of any opportunity they get to eat. For civilians, though, meal timing can be more structured.

Having five to six small meals throughout the day, as opposed to three large ones, can help stabilize blood sugar levels, boosting energy, and ensuring the body is consistently supplied with the nutrients it needs.

Although the nutritional needs of soldiers and civilians differ significantly, there are many transferable principles. Adopting the best combat nutrition practices can supplement your fitness regimen and facilitate better recovery. By integrating these lessons into your everyday routine, you can transform into your version of a wellness warrior. No war required.

Chapter 11. Creating Your Personal Combat Nutrition Plan

Creating your personal Combat Nutrition Plan is a strategic process, an interweaving of knowledge about military nourishments with your own individual fitness goals and routines. Let's start with understanding the basic principles behind military eating habits and the nutritional science that fuels these warriors.

11.1. Military Eating Habits and Nutritional Science

For a soldier, survival is critical and the food they consume prepares their body to withstand extreme conditions. The rations in the field are known as Meals, Ready-to-Eat (MRE). Each MRE provides an average of 1250 kilocalories, rich in protein and carbohydrates to maximize the body's performance and endurance levels. This meal plan can be a guideline for athletes and individuals attentive to their fitness.

While designing your Combat Nutrition Plan, keep in mind to:

- Prioritize protein: Soldiers require proteins in abundance for muscle repair, growth, and maintenance. Similarly, high-intensity workouts can cause muscle tearing that demands adequate protein for repair.

- Power up with carbohydrates: Soldiers load up on carbohydrates to fuel their bodies for rigorous activities. Carbs convert swiftly into glucose, providing immediate energy.

- Don't forget the fats: While fats are generally frowned upon, healthy fats are important soldiers' diets to retain energy reserves when carbohydrates run out.

Drawing from soldiers' dietary habits, it's clear an ideal Combat Nutrition Plan would require a balanced intake of these three macronutrients. Understand your body's calorie requirements and meal scheduling for optimal performance.

11.2. Individual Calorie Requirements and Meal Scheduling

Your Combat Nutrition Plan is not a one-size-fits-all template. It has to be tailored to suit your age, gender, weight, height, and especially your physical activity level. A comprehensive study of your calorie intake and energy expenditure is crucial.

Maintain a calorific diary, logging the caloric value of every food item you consume for a week. To compute your baseline calorie requirement, you can opt for online tools. The number obtained can either be reduced for weight loss, increased for muscle gain, or maintained for balanced weight.

Soldiers eat their meals at regular intervals to prevent a drop in energy levels and cognitive function. Similarly, athletes are encouraged to eat every 2-3 hours, but on a much smaller scale –think of them as 'mini-meals'. Design your Combat Nutrition Plan with 5-6 meals a day, ensuring a regular energy supply to your body and curbing unnecessary hunger.

11.3. Developing the Combat Nutrition Plan

Now that we've understood the basics let's dive into the development of your personalized Combat Nutrition Plan.

1. Asses your Goals: Identify what you wish to achieve from this plan –muscle gain, fat loss, or weight maintenance.

2. Calculate your Macronutrients: According to the goals identified, set the ratio of carbs, proteins, and fats you need in your diet.

3. Choose your Foods Wisely: Incorporate a range of lean proteins, complex carbs, and healthy fats in your diet. It can include lean meats, whole grains, fruits, vegetables, nuts, and seeds.

4. Plan your Meals: Break down your daily macros across each meal – making sure to include proteins in each. Schedule meals around your workout regime – load up on carbs before and after a workout, and intake proteins after.

5. Hydrate: Soldiers are well aware of the importance of hydration. Ensure you drink an adequate amount of water daily.

11.4. The Importance of Flexibility and Adaptation

Remember, this Combat Nutrition Plan is not definitive. Monitor results every few weeks, revising the plan if you're not achieving your set weight or fitness goals. It's important to adapt to see progress. Soldiers induct new techniques, change tactics, and adapt in the face of adversity. Similarly, you should be willing to tweak your plan, change your meals, or increase/decrease your caloric intake and macronutrient ratio.

The military strategies and nutrition tips woven into this chapter not only guide athletes and fitness enthusiasts towards their goals but also offer lifestyle lessons in discipline, organization, and resilience, necessary components of soldiering. The personalized Combat Nutrition Plan aims to fuse the virtue of this soldier-stance into your everyday life. By adhering to it, you are cultivating a sound mind and body, transforming yourself into a fortress of wellness and strength.

Chapter 12. Combat Nutrition Recipes: From the Mess Hall to Your Kitchen

Ready to take a step closer to absolute fitness and resilience with a military-grade diet? With these recipes originating straight from the mess hall, you can bring the proven benefits of combat nutrition right into your kitchen.

Let's march into what we have in store for you!

12.1. Ingredients with a Purpose

First, it's crucial to understand that in combat nutrition, every ingredient has a purpose. The meals aren't haphazard combinations of food, but fine-tuned formulas that target enhanced energy, endurance, recovery, and overall health.

1. **Protein:** This primary building block of muscle comes from lean meats, fish, eggs, and plant sources such as beans and lentils.

2. **Carbohydrates:** These are the body's first line of energy and come from grains, fruits, and starchy vegetables.

3. **Healthy Fats:** Unsaturated fats should be included for heart and brain health. Avocados, olive oil, eggs, and fish are great sources.

4. **Vitamins and Minerals:** A variety of produce ensures the body receives essential nutrients for various functions, like immune response and energy metabolism.

5. **Hydration:** This is a cornerstone for peak performance—not just water, but electrolyte-rich fluids with salts and sugars, like coconut water and sports drinks.

Now, let's dive into the heart of the kitchen battlefield, where you'll learn how to combine these ingredients for delicious, performance-enhancing meals!

12.2. Combat Breakfast: Sunrise Fuel-Up

Fuel your morning with this protein-packed breakfast, which contains a balanced blend of energizing nutrients to kick-start your day.

1. **1 cup plain rolled oats**
2. **3 tablespoons of almond butter**
3. **1 medium banana, sliced**
4. **1 tablespoon chia seeds**
5. **2 egg whites**
6. **1 cup almond milk**
7. **1 scoop protein powder (either whey or plant-based)**
8. **A pinch of salt, cinnamon, and sweetener to taste**

Combine the oats and almond milk in a pot, bringing to a boil and then reducing to simmer until creamy. Stir in the protein powder, chia seeds, almond butter, and seasoning. Cook the egg whites separately and place them on top. Add your banana slices, and your sunrise fuel-up is ready to be served!

12.3. Midday Meals: Stamina-Boosting Lunch

Create a powerhouse salad that's teeming with nutrients to nourish you throughout the day.

1. **2 cups mixed greens**

2. **1 cup cooked quinoa**

3. **1/2 cup chickpeas**

4. **1 grilled chicken breast, sliced**

5. **1/2 medium avocado, sliced**

6. **1 small diced bell pepper**

7. **A sprinkle of nuts or seeds**

8. **Your choice of low-fat dressing**

Combine all ingredients in a large salad bowl, tossing gently to mix. Opt for a dash of balsamic vinaigrette or lemon juice and olive oil mix as your dressing.

12.4. Fortified Dinner: Recovery Feast

This hearty meal delivers protein, fiber, healthy fats and carbs, helping your body repair and recover post-workout.

1. **1 salmon fillet**

2. **1 cup cooked brown rice**

3. **1 cup steamed broccoli**

4. **1 tablespoon olive oil**

5. **Lemon, salt, and pepper to taste**

Bake the salmon at 375°F (190°C) for 20 minutes, seasoning with olive oil, lemon, salt, and pepper. Serve with the steamed broccoli and cooked brown rice on the side.

Interchanging your culinary choices while keeping in mind the balance of nutrients is key to sustaining this healthy, resilient lifestyle, just like our men and women on the battlefield.

Next, we step into hydration, an essential realm in combat nutrition, often underplayed.

12.5. Hydration: Sustaining the Flow

Not all fluids hydrate you the same way. Due to constant sweating and vigorous activity, our military heroes need something more potent than water—they need electrolytes. You can prepare this homemade electrolyte drink:

1. **4 cups water**

2. **1/2 teaspoon salt**

3. **5 tablespoons honey**

4. **1 cup orange juice**

5. **1/2 cup lemon juice**

Combine all ingredients, stirring until the salt and honey dissolve. Chill in the refrigerator and consume during your workout or active periods in the day.

Remember, the discipline and strength of our soldiers stem from a well-balanced and nourishing diet. Unswerving commitment to health and fitness matters as much on your home turf as it does in a combat zone.

Start your combat fitness journey today, and see the transformative power of military nutrition unfold with every meal you make!

* 9 7 9 8 8 5 7 5 1 7 5 0 5 *